Air Fryer Recipes
For Diabetics

Control Diabetes and Live Well

With Delicious Easy-to-Make Recipes

Lilith Ballard

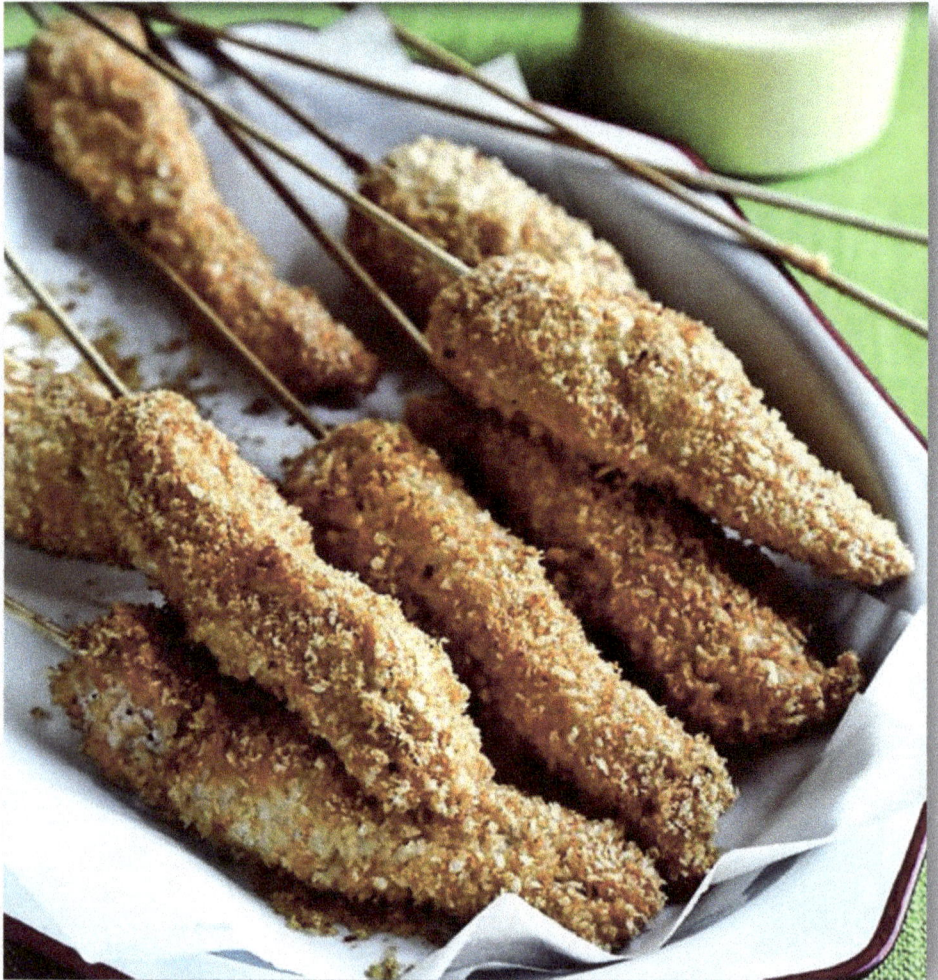

professional before attempting any techniques outlined in this book.

by reading this document, the reader agrees that under no circumstances is the author responsible for any losses, direct or indirect, which are incurred as a result of the use of information contained within this document, including, but not limited to, — errors, omissions, or inaccuracies.

Table of Contents

AIR-FRIED CINNAMON BISCUIT BITE

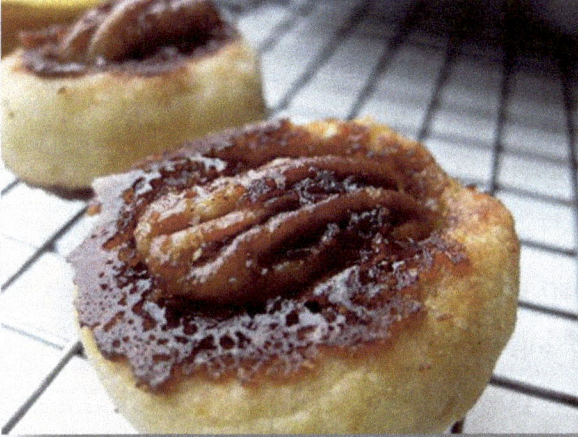

Preparation Time: 25 minutes

Cooking Time: 16 minutes

Servings: 8

Nutritional values:

- Calories: 325 kcal
- Fat: 7 g

- Carbohydrates: 1 g
- Proteins: 8 g

Ingredients:

- 2/3 cup all-purpose flour
- 2/3 cup whole-wheat flour
- ¼ tsp. ground cinnamon
- ¼ tsp. kosher salt
- 1/3 cup whole milk
- 1 tsp. baking powder
- 4 tbsp. cold salted butter
- Cooking spray
- 2 cups powdered sugar
- 3 tbsp. water

Directions:

1. Cut the cold salted butter into small pieces. Add salt, cinnamon, baking powder, and flour together in a bowl, and whisk them together. Add butter to the mixture and stir it until the mixture is even.

2. Add milk to the mixture, and stir it together until it forms dough balls. Knead the dough on a surface that has some flour. Prepare smooth and cohesive balls. This should take half a minute.

3. Now, you can cut the dough into 16 pieces and gently roll each of them into a smooth ball.

4. Coat air fryer basket with cooking spray. Then, you can cook the dough at 350°F until it puffs up and goes brown. The cooking should be for about 10 to 12 minutes.

5. Now, you can remove the doughnut balls and place them on a wire rack over a foil. Do the same with the other dough balls.

6. To serve people who are not diabetic, you can mix some granulated sugar with water and sprinkle the solution on the doughnut balls.

AIR-FRIED SPICY CHICKEN WING DRUMETTES

Preparation Time: 15 minutes

Cooking Time: 28 minutes

Servings: 2

Nutritional values:

- Calories: 488 kcal
- Fat: 30 g
- Carbohydrates: 20 g
- Proteins: 25 g

Ingredients:

- Cooking spray
- 3/8 tsp. crushed red pepper
- 3 tbsp. honey
- 2 tbsp. unsalted chicken stock
- 2 tbsp. chopped unsalted roasted peanuts
- 10 large chicken drumettes

- ¼ cup rice vinegar
- 1 tbsp. toasted sesame oil
- 1 tbsp. lower-sodium soy sauce
- 1 finely chopped garlic clove
- 1 tbsp. chopped fresh chives

Directions:

1. The first step is to place the chicken in the basket of your air fryer. Spray cooking spray on them. Cook them for about 25 minutes at the temperature of 400°F. By then, the chicken will be crispy. Remember to turn them over halfway into the cooking time.

2. While the chicken is being cooked, mix the garlic, crushed red pepper, soy sauce, oil, stock, honey, and vinegar together in a skillet.

3. Heat them with medium-high heat for the mixture to simmer. Wait until the sauce thickens slightly. It will feel like syrup. This will happen within only 6 minutes of heating.

4. Now, you can place the chicken drumettes in a bowl and add the honey syrup mixture to the drumettes.

5. Toss them to get the chicken coated.

6. Sprinkle them with chives and peanuts before they are served. This dish is best eaten hot or warm.

SWEET POTATO CHIPS

Preparation Time: 5 minutes

Cooking Time: 55 minutes

Servings: 4

Nutritional values:

- Calories: 60 kcal
- Fat: 3.5 g
- Carbohydrates: 2 g
- Proteins: 1 g

Ingredients:

- Cooking spray
- ¼ tsp. sea salt
- ¼ tsp. freshly ground black pepper
- 1 tsp. chopped fresh rosemary (optional)
- 1 tbsp. canola oil
- 1 medium sweet potato

Directions:

1. Cut the potatoes into 1/8-inch-thick slices.

2. Get a big bowl. Pour some cold water in it. Soak the slices of potatoes in the water and leave it for 20 minutes.

3. Drain the potatoes and pat them dry with a paper towel.

4. Clean the bowl before adding the rosemary, pepper, salt, and oil into it. Of course, you need to add the potatoes to the mixture and toss them together.

5. Apply some cooking spray on your air fryer basket. Then, divide the slices of potatoes into two parts.

6. Cook the first part in your air fryer at 350°F. Cook it for about a quarter of an hour. By then, it will be done and crispy. Ensure you check it every 5 minutes.

7. Remove the first batch and start with the second batch.

8. Put them on a plate and allow them cool for 5 minutes before you serve them. On the other hand, if your guests are not around, you can keep the potatoes in an airtight container to keep them warm.

CRISPY TOASTED SESAME TOFU

Preparation Time: 5 minutes

Cooking Time: 60 minutes

Servings: 4

Nutritional values:

- Calories: 445 kcal
- Fat: 20 g
- Carbohydrates: 12 g
- Proteins: 23 g

Ingredients:

- Cooking spray
- 2 tbsp. lower-sodium soy sauce
- 2 tbsp. chopped scallions
- 2 packs extra-firm tofu
- 2 packs boil-in-bag brown rice
- ¼ cup fresh orange juice (from 1 orange)

- ½ tsp. kosher salt
- ½ tsp. cornstarch
- 1 tsp. rice vinegar
- 1 tbsp. toasted sesame seeds
- 1 tbsp. and 1 tsp. toasted sesame oil
- 1 tbsp. and 1 tsp. honey

Directions:

1. Drain and cut the tofu into 1-inch cubes. Preheat your oven to 200°F.

2. Line a plate with a paper towel and place the cubes of tofu on the plate. Cover it with another layer of paper towels before covering everything with another plate.

3. Leave it like that for half an hour before you coat the tofu with cooking spray.

4. Place the tofu in your air fryer basket. Place half in a single layer. So, all the tofu cubes will be on two layers.

5. Cook it at 375°F for a quarter of an hour. After 7 to 8 minutes, you can turn the cubes over. When they are done, they'll be crispy and golden brown in color.

6. Remove them and keep them warm in your preheated oven.

7. Whisk the cornstarch, rice vinegar, sesame oil, honey, soy sauce, and orange juice together and heat the mixture on high heat. Continue heating and whisking it until it starts

to boil. Whisk it a little further until it becomes thicker. This should not take you more than 3 minutes.

8.   Prepare the rice and add some salt. Add the tofu to the soy sauce mixture. Serve the rice and add some tofu before you sprinkle the dish with some sesame seeds and scallions.

AIR-FRIED FLAXSEED FRENCH TOAST STICKS WITH BERRIES

Preparation Time: 21 minutes

Cooking Time: 10-20 minutes

Servings: 4

Nutritional values:

- Calories: 361 kcal
- Fat: 10 g
- Carbohydrates: 5 g
- Proteins: 14 g

Ingredients:

- Cooking spray
- 8 tsp. pure maple syrup, divided
- 4 whole-grain bread slices
- 2/3 cup flaxseed meal
- 2 large eggs

- 2 cups sliced fresh strawberries
- ¼ cup reduced-fat milk
- ½ tsp. ground cinnamon
- 1 tsp. vanilla extract

Directions:

1. Divide each slice of bread into 4 sticks. Mix the cinnamon, vanilla, milk, and eggs together in a small bowl.
2. Place the flaxseed meal in another bowl. Soak the pieces of bread in the egg mixture, one piece at a time. Then, transfer the soaked sticks of bread to the flaxseed meal for coating.
3. After that, you need to coat the breadsticks with cooking spray.
4. Arrange the sticks of bread in your air fryer basket, but make sure there are spaces between them.
5. Cook them at 375°F for just 5 minutes. You can turn them over before you cook them for another 5 minutes. They should be crunchy and golden brown by then.
6. Place them on a plate, top the sticks of bread with ½ cup of strawberries and 2 tsp. of maple syrup, and serve them.

BEET CHIPS

Preparation Time: 5 minutes

Cooking Time: 60 minutes

Servings: 4

Nutritional values:

- Calories: 47 kcal
- Fat: 2 g
- Carbohydrates: 0.2 g
- Proteins: 1 g

Ingredients:

- 3/4 tsp. kosher salt
- 3 medium-size red beets
- 2 tsp. canola oil
- ¼ tsp. black pepper

Directions:

1. Peel the beets and cut them into 1/8-inch-thick slices.

2. Add oil, pepper, and salt to the beets, and toss the mixture together.

3. Divide the beets into two portions and cook one portion first.

4. Cook half portion in your air fryer at 320°F for about 30 minutes. Don't forget to shake your air fryer basket every 5 minutes.

5. Do the same with the second portion. You can now serve them in four plates for different people.

SWEET POTATO CRISPS

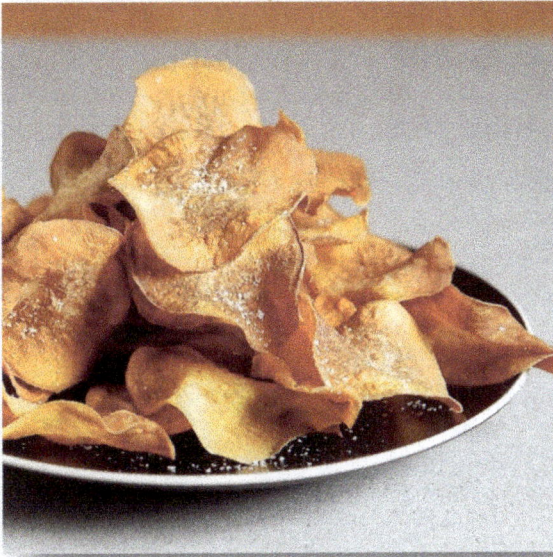

Preparation Time: 5 minutes

Cooking Time: 30 minutes

Servings: 8

Nutritional values:

- Calories: 122

- Fat: 6 g
- Carbohydrates: 15 g
- Proteins: 1 g

Ingredients:

- 2 large sweet potatoes, shaved thin using mandolin
- Spanish paprika and sea salt to taste

Dips, optional:

- ¼ cup cashew cheese
- ¼ cup spinach walnut pesto

Directions:

1. Preheat Air Fryer to 330°F.
2. Place sweet potatoes flat on baking sheets with spaces in between pieces. Drizzle in oil; season lightly with paprika and sea salt.
3. Put baking sheet inside the air fryer basket. Fry for 30 minutes. Cool completely to room temperature before serving. Serve with cashew cheese and spinach walnut pesto.

SCRAMBLED SALMON EGG

Preparation Time: 6 minutes

Cooking Time: 22 minutes

Servings: 2

Nutritional values:

- Calories: 120 kcal
- Fat: 4.5 g
- Carbohydrates: 13 g
- Proteins: 9.9 g

Ingredients:

- 2 eggs
- 1 piece smoked salmon
- 1 small red onion
- 2 tsp. olive oil
- 1/3 cup milk, low fat
- ¼ tsp. black pepper
- 2 tbsp. fresh dill

Directions:

1. Preheat the Air Fryer to 330°F.

2. In a skillet, heat the oil. Sauté onions until translucent. Set aside.

3. Meanwhile, in a bowl, combine milk, eggs, salmon, and pepper.

4. Place the salmon mixture inside the basket. Scramble the eggs until set.

5. Sprinkle dill all over. Serve.

FRIED GREEN TOMATOES

Preparation Time: 8 minutes

Cooking Time: 15-20 minutes

Servings: 2

Nutritional values:

- Calories: 60 kcal
- Carbohydrates: 5 g
- Fat: 3.2 g
- Proteins: 3.6 g

Ingredients:

- 2 green tomatoes, sliced into ¼ inch thick
- 1 cup buttermilk
- 1 cup panko bread crumbs
- ½ cup almond flour
- 1 tsp. salt
- ½ tbsp. Creole seasoning
- ½ tsp. pepper

Directions:

1. Slice the tomatoes to ¼-inch thickness. Sprinkle both sides with salt and pepper.

2. Put the buttermilk, flour, and the mixture of panko crumbs and Creole seasoning in 3 different shallow containers. Dredge each slice of tomato in the flour.

3. Dip it into the buttermilk and coat it with the panko mixture. Gently press the coating to make them stick.

4. Put the rack in the cooking basket of the Air Fryer. Arrange 3 coated tomato slices on top of the rack and spray with non-stick cooking spray. Set the fryer to 400°F and cook for 5 minutes. Transfer the cooked tomatoes to a platter and cook the rest of the coated tomato slices.

5. Sprinkle the cooked tomatoes with a little creole seasoning and serve them with ranch dressing.

TUNA SANDWICH

Preparation Time: 9 minutes

Cooking Time: 10-15 minutes

Servings: 2

Nutritional values:

- Calories: 160
- Fat: 10 g
- Carbohydrates: 14 g
- Proteins: 24 g

Ingredients:

- 1 5-ounce can solid white tuna in water, drained
- 2 slices wheat bread
- 1 tsp. onion, chopped finely
- 1 celery stalk, chopped finely
- 2 tbsp. mayonnaise, low fat
- 4 slices ripe tomato
- ½ cup sharp cheddar cheese, reduced-fat, shredded

- 1/8 tsp. celery salt
- Pinch black pepper

Directions:

1. Put the bread slices in the cooking basket. Set the Air Fryer to 400°F and cook for 3 minutes.

2. In a bowl, combine the mayonnaise, tuna, salt, pepper, onion, and celery. Divide the mixture and spread in the 2 toasted bread slices. Put 2 slices of tomato and cheese on top of each bread slice. Put one sandwich in the cooking basket at a time.

3. Set the Air Fryer to 400 degrees and cook for 4 minutes. Cook the other sandwich.

MUSHROOM FRITTATA

Preparation Time: 7 minutes

Cooking Time: 26 minutes

Servings: 4

Nutritional values:

- Calories: 129
- Fat: 17.8 g
- Carbohydrates: 15.4 g
- Proteins: 17.6 g

Ingredients:

- 2 eggs
- ½ cup fresh mushrooms, sliced
- 1 tbsp. olive oil
- 1 Roma tomato, halved
- Pinch salt
- Pinch ground black pepper

Directions:

1. Set the Air Fryer to 400°F.

2. Sautee the mushrooms until cooked through. Season the mushrooms with salt and pepper to taste. Once cooked, transfer to a plate and set aside.

3. Cook tomato. The tomatoes will become tender when ready. Sprinkle salt and pepper on the tomatoes. Transfer them to a plate once they are cooked.

4. Cook eggs the way you prefer. For an English breakfast, eggs are usually either fried or scrambled.

5. Arrange the mushrooms, tomato, and eggs on your plate. Serve.

AVOCADO TACO FRY

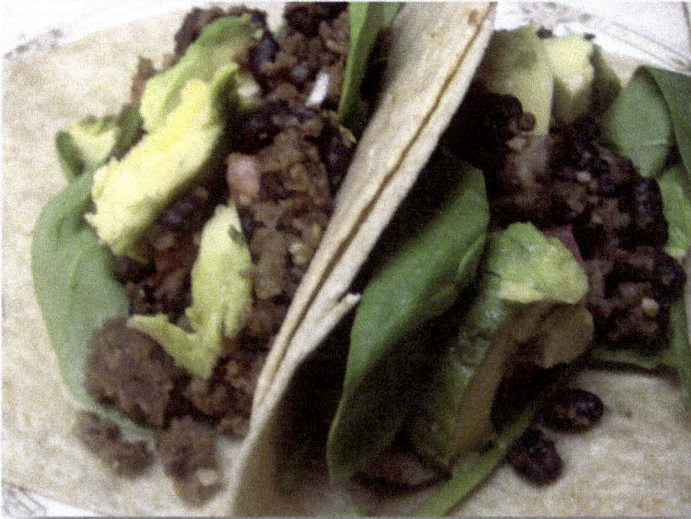

Preparation Time: 6 minutes

Cooking Time: 28 minutes

Servings: 4

Nutritional values:

- Calories: 140 kcal
- Fat: 8.8 g
- Carbohydrates: 12 g
- Proteins: 6 g

Ingredients:

- 1 avocado
- 1 egg
- ½ cup panko bread crumbs
- Salt, to taste
- Tortillas and toppings

Directions:

1. Remove the flesh from each of the avocado shells and slice them into wedges.
2. Beat the egg in a shallow bowl and put the breadcrumbs in another bowl. Dip the avocado into the bowl with the beaten egg and coat with the breadcrumbs. Sprinkle the coated wedges with a bit of salt.
3. Arrange them in the cooking basket in a single layer.
4. Set the Air Fryer to 392°F and cook for 15 minutes. Shake the basket halfway through the cooking process.
5. Put them on tortillas with your preferred toppings.

BLUEBERRY CREAM CHEESE SANDWICH

Preparation Time: 9 minutes

Cooking Time: 10-15 minutes

Servings: 4

Nutritional values:

- Calories: 70 kcal
- Fat: 4.5 g
- Carbohydrates: 6 g
- Proteins: 2 g

Ingredients:

- 4 slices wheat bread
- ¼ cup fresh blueberries
- 1 ½ cups corn flakes, crumbled
- 4 tbsp. whipped cream cheese, berry-flavored
- 2 eggs, beaten
- 2 tsp. Stevia

- 1/3 cup milk, low fat
- ¼ tsp. salt
- ¼ tsp. ground nutmeg

Directions:

1. Preheat the Air Fryer to 400°F.
2. Put the eggs, salt, sugar, nutmeg, and milk in a bowl. Mix well.
3. In another bowl, mix the whipped cream cheese and blueberries.
4. Slit the top part of the crust of each bread slice. Fill each slice with 2 tbsp. of the berry mixture. Soak the stuffed bread slices in the egg mixture until completely covered.
5. Coat them with corn flakes and press to make them stick. Put the coated bread slices in the cooking basket of the Air Fryer. Cook for 8 minutes.
6. Serve while hot.

AIR FRYER BAKED POTATO

Preparation Time: 2 minutes

Cooking Time: 35-40 minutes

Servings: 3

Nutritional values:

- Calories: 213 kcal
- Fat: 4 g
- Proteins: 4 g
- Carbohydrates: 39 g

Ingredients:

- 3 Idaho or Russet Baking Potatoes
- 1 to 2 tbsp. olive oil
- 1 tsp. parsley
- 1 tbsp. garlic
- 1 tbsp. salt

Directions:

1. Wash the potatoes very well.

2. Poke several holes in the potatoes with a fork.

3. Sprinkle the potatoes with olive oil. Evenly rub the potatoes with parsley, garlic, and salt.

4. Arrange the potatoes in the air fryer basket and cook for 35 to 40 minutes at 392°F until fork tender.

5. Serve with your favorite dipping, sour cream, or fresh parsley.

AIR FRYER MEXICAN STREET CORN

Preparation Time: 8 minutes

Cooking Time: 15-20 minutes

Servings: 4

Nutritional values:

- Calories: 102 kcal
- Fat: 3 g
- Carbohydrates: 17 g
- Proteins: 4 g

Ingredients:

- 4 pieces fresh corn on the cob
- ¼ cup crumbled Feta cheese or cotija cheese
- ¼ cup chopped fresh cilantro
- ½ tsp. Stone House Seasoning or Mrs. Dash Southwest Chipotle Seasoning

- ¼ tsp. chili powder
- 1 medium lime cut into wedges

Directions:

1. Arrange the corn in the basket of air fryer. Cook at 390°For ten minutes.
2. While cooking, sprinkle the cheese all over the corn, and cook for another five minutes at 390°F.
3. Quickly remove corn from the air fryer.
4. Sprinkle on top with Stone House or Mrs. Dash seasoning, cilantro, and chili powder.
5. Serve corn with lime wedges alongside.

AIR FRYER CORN ON THE COB

Preparation Time: 6 minutes

Cooking Time: 15-20 minutes

Servings: 2

Nutritional values:

- Calories: 140 kcal
- Fat: 7.8 g
- Proteins: 3 g
- Carbohydrates: 18 g

Ingredients:

- 2 ears fresh sweet corn husk
- 1 tbsp. oil
- Pinch salt
- Dash pepper

Directions:

1.   Remove silk of corn and cut in half to yield four pieces.

2.   Slowly pour 1 tbsp. of oil all over the corn and spread by rubbing with your hands.

3.   Arrange the corn halves in the air fryer basket. Cook for eight minutes at 380°F.

4.   When the fryer strikes at the exactly four-minute mark, quickly remove the basket and shake, and then return to the fryer to continue cooking for the remaining 4 minutes.

5.   Remove the corn from the basket when the timer is up. Sprinkle with additional pepper and salt if desired.

6.   Serve hot.

AIR FRYER TACO BELL CRUNCH WRAP

Preparation Time: 11 minutes

Cooking Time: 18 minutes

Servings: 6

Nutritional values:

- Calories: 954 kcal
- Fat: 30 g
- Proteins: 42 g
- Carbohydrates: 19 g

Ingredients:

- 2 pounds ground beef
- 1 1/3 cups water
- 2 servings Homemade Taco Seasoning, see accompanying recipe below
- 6 large 12-inch flour tortillas
- 12 ounces nacho cheese

- 3 roma tomatoes
- 2 cup shredded lettuce
- 2 cups sour cream
- 2 cups Mexican blend cheese
- 6 tostada shell
- Cooking Spray

For Homemade Taco Seasoning:

- 1 ½ tbsp. ground cumin
- 1 tbsp. chili powder
- 1 tsp. garlic powder
- 1 tsp. paprika
- 1 tsp. salt
- 1 tsp. onion powder
- ½ tsp. dried oregano
- 1 tsp. black pepper

Directions:

1. Preheat the air fryer at 400°F.
2. Cook the ground beef in a skillet on medium heat until the pink color has disappeared.
3. Stir in two servings of the homemade taco seasoning and 1 ½ cups water; bring to a boil. Reduce heat and cook the beef in a simmer until it thickens. Set aside.

4. Spread each flour tortilla on a large plate and fill with 2/3 cups of cooked beef, 4 tbsp. nacho cheese, 1/3 cup sour cream, 1 tostada, 1/3 cup lettuce, 1/6th roma tomatoes and 1/3 cup cheese.

5. Seal the taco bell by folding the edges up and over the center to resemble a pinwheel. Repeat the steps with the remaining wraps.

6. Spray the fry basket with oil.

7. Arrange the taco bell, seam side down in the fryer and spray with oil. Cook for two minutes until golden brown.

8. Gently flip the taco bell with a spatula and spray with oil. Cook for two minutes longer and repeat with the rest of the wraps. Let cool for a minute.

9. For Homemade Taco Seasoning:

10. Combine all taco seasoning ingredients in a bowl. Transfer to an airtight container and store in a dry, dark place.

CRISPY VEGGIE FRIES

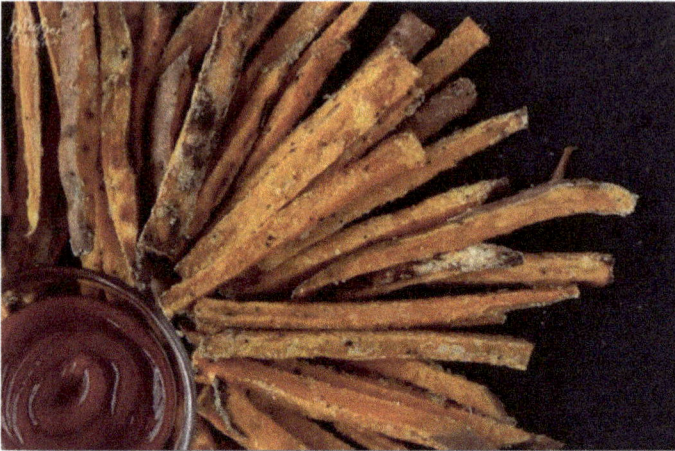

Preparation Time: 6 minutes

Cooking Time: 10-15 minutes

Servings: 6

Nutritional values:

- Calories: 229 kcal
- Fat: 1.6 g
- Carbohydrates: 45.5 g
- Proteins: 7.8 g

Ingredients:

- 1 cup rice flour
- 2 tbsp. Follow Your Heart Vegan Egg powder*
- 2 tbsp. nutritional yeast flakes, divided
- 1 cup panko bread crumbs (gluten-free or regular)
- 2/3 cup cold water
- Pinch salt
- Dash pepper
- Assorted vegetables (green beans, cauliflower, zucchini, or cauliflower)

Directions:

1. Cut assorted veggies into French fry shapes or bite-size chunks.
2. Pour the rice flour into a shallow dish.
3. Whisk together in another shallow dish the Vegan Egg powder, 2/3 cup of water and 1 tbsp. Nutritional yeast flakes until smooth.
4. Combine in a separate shallow dish the panko breadcrumbs, 1 tbsp. Nutritional yeast, salt, and pepper.
5. Dip each vegetable in the rice flour, and then dip in the Vegan Egg mixture, and lastly in the breadcrumb mixture.
6. Press the vegetable to coat well. Repeat the steps until all the vegetables are coated.

7. Lightly mist your air fryer basket or line your baking sheet with parchment and then spray more oil.

8. Gently load the veggie fries into the basket and spray a little amount of oil.

9. Cook the veggie fries for eight minutes at 380°F until crisp-golden.

10. Serve!

AIR FRYER SOFT PRETZELS

Preparation Time: 9 minutes

Cooking Time: 18 minutes

Servings: 12

Nutritional values:

- Calories: 214 kcal
- Fat: 4.7 g
- Carbohydrates: 17 g
- Proteins: 5.3 g

Ingredients:

- 1 ½ cups warm
- 2 tsp. kosher salt
- 1 tbsp. sugar
- 1 package active dry yeast
- 2 ounces melted butter
- 4 ½ cups all-purpose flour
- 2/3 cup baking soda
- 10 cups water

- 1 egg yolk
- Pretzel salt

Directions:

1. In a bowl of your stand mixer fitted with a dough hook, mix the water, salt, and sugar together. Sprinkle on top with yeast and let sit for five minutes.

2. Pour the flour into the bowl and add the butter; combine the mixture together at low speed.

3. Increase the speed to medium and knead the dough for 5 minutes until smooth and does not stick to the side of the bowl.

4. Transfer the dough to a greased bowl; cover with plastic wrap. Let dough sit for 50 to 60 minutes at a warm temperature until the size has doubled.

5. Prepare two baking sheets and line them with parchment paper and then mist with nonstick spray.

6. Heat up your air fryer at 400°F.

7. Meanwhile, combine in a large roasting pan or stockpot the baking soda and 10 cups of water; bring to a boil.

8. Lay the pretzel dough on a greased work surface and equally divide into 12 pieces. Roll each dough piece into an 18" rope and then twist to form into a pretzel shape.

9. Working on each piece of pretzel, place in the boiling water for thirty seconds and quickly remove from water. Transfer the pretzels to the prepared baking sheet.

10. Beat the egg yolk in 1 tbsp. of water and brush over the pretzels.

11. Sprinkle the pretzels with pretzel salt and load about 3 to 4 pieces into the air fryer basket. Cook for 6 minutes at 400°F; turn over and cook for additional 6 minutes or until dark golden brown.

12. Serve!

AIR FRYER BLACKBERRY HAND PIES

Preparation Time: 11 minutes

Cooking Time: 13 minutes

Servings: 6

Nutritional values:

- Calories :292 kcal
- Fat: 8 g
- Carbohydrates: 21 g
- Proteins: 3 g

Ingredients:

- 1 package refrigerated pie dough
- 1 beaten egg

For the filling:

- 12 ounces fresh blackberries
- 3 tbsp. all-purpose flour

- ¼ cup sugar

- ½ tsp. cinnamon

- 2 tbsp. lemon juice

For the icing:

- 1 cup powdered sugar

- ½ lemon

Directions:

1. Preheat your air fryer.
2. For the filling:
3. Wash the blackberries in running water. Transfer to a plate lined with a paper towel to drain excess water. Let it sit for one hour to dry completely.
4. Cut the fruits in half and transfer to a medium-sized bowl.
5. Add the sugar, flour, cinnamon, and lemon juice to the bowl with strawberries, tossing to combine well.
6. Pour the blackberry mixture into a medium-sized pot and cook on medium heat.
7. Using a potato masher, mash the berries until somewhat chunky. Turn off heat.
8. Set aside.
9. For the pie:
10. Dust the countertop with flour and lay the pie crusts on top. Roll the crusts out to ¼-inch thickness.

11.   Cut out six circles from the crusts using a large circle cutter. Arrange the dough circles on a baking sheet.

12.   Fill the dough with one tbsp. filling and brush the sides with beaten egg.

13.   Fold the pie dough over, pressing down with your fingers to seal tightly. Leave indentations on the sides of the dough by pressing the edges with fork tines.

14.   Using a pastry brush, lightly paint the top of the pies with beaten egg and lightly sprinkle with sugar.

15.   Cook two pieces of pie dough at a time in the air fryer for 8 to 10 minutes at 380°F or until flaky and golden brown.

16.   For the icing:

17.   Put the sugar and lemon in a small bowl, whisking until combined. Slightly cool and top the hand pies with an icing drizzle.

18.   Serve!

PORK, BEEF AND LAMB RECIPES

PORK TRINOZA WRAPPED IN HAM

Preparation Time: 8 minutes

Cooking Time: 10-15 minutes

Servings: 6

Nutritional values:

- Calories: 282
- Fat: 23.41 g
- Carbohydrates: 0 g
- Proteins: 16.59 g

Ingredients:

- 6 pieces Serrano ham, thinly sliced
- 454 g pork, halved, with butter and crushed
- 6 g salt
- 1 g black pepper

- 227 g fresh spinach leaves, divided
- 4 slices mozzarella cheese, divided
- 18 g sun-dried tomatoes, divided
- 10 ml olive oil, divided

Directions:

1. Place 3 pieces of ham on baking paper, slightly overlapping each other. Place 1 half of the pork in the ham. Repeat with the other half.
2. Season the inside of the pork rolls with salt and pepper.
3. Place half of the spinach, cheese, and sun-dried tomatoes on top of the pork loin, leaving a 13 mm border on all sides.
4. Roll the fillet around the filling well and tie it with a kitchen cord to keep it closed.
5. Repeat the process for the other pork steak and place them in the fridge.
6. Select Preheat in the air fryer and press Start/Pause.
7. Brush 5 ml of olive oil on each wrapped steak and place them in the preheated air fryer.
8. Select Steak. Set the timer to 9 minutes and press Start/Pause.
9. Allow it to cool for 10 minutes before cutting.

STUFFED CABBAGE AND PORK LOIN ROLLS

Preparation Time: 5 minutes

Cooking Time: 28 minutes

Servings: 4

Nutritional values:

- Calories: 120 kcal
- Fat: 3.41 g
- Carbohydrates: 0 g
- Proteins: 20.99 g

Ingredients:

- 500 g white cabbage
- 1 onion
- 8 pork tenderloin steaks
- 2 carrots
- 4 tbsp. soy sauce
- 50 g olive oil

- Salt
- 8 sheets rice

Directions:

1. Put the chopped cabbage in the Thermo mix glass together with the onion and the chopped carrot.

2. Select 5 seconds, speed 5. Add the extra virgin olive oil. Select 5 minutes, left turn, spoon speed.

3. Cut the tenderloin steaks into thin strips. Add the meat to the Thermomix glass. Select 5 minutes, varoma temperature, left turn, spoon speed. Without beaker

4. Add the soy sauce. Select 5 minutes, varoma temperature, left turn, spoon speed. Rectify salt. Let it cold down.

5. Hydrate the rice slices. Extend and distribute the filling between them.

6. Make the rolls, folding so that the edges are completely closed. Place the rolls in the air fryer and paint with the oil.

7. Select 10 minutes, 180°C.

HOMEMADE FLAMINGOS

Preparation Time: 8 minutes

Cooking Time: 10-15 minutes

Servings: 4

Nutritional values:

- Calories: 482 kcal
- Fat: 23.41 g
- Carbohydrates: 0 g
- Proteins: 16.59 g

Ingredients:

- 400 g very thin sliced pork fillets c / n
- 2 boiled and chopped eggs
- 100 g chopped Serrano ham
- 1 beaten egg
- Breadcrumbs

Directions:

1. Make a roll with the pork fillets. Introduce half-cooked egg and Serrano ham. So that the roll does not lose its shape, fasten with a string or chopsticks.

2. Pass the rolls through the beaten egg and then through the breadcrumbs until it forms a good layer.

3. Preheat the air fryer for a few minutes at 180°C.

4. Insert the rolls in the basket and set the timer for about 8 minutes at 180°C.

BEEF SCALLOPS

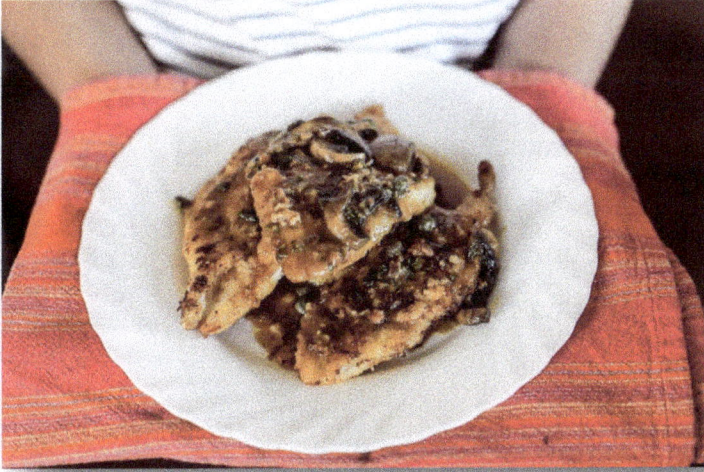

Preparation Time: 9 minutes

Cooking Time: 27 minutes

Servings: 4

Nutritional values:

- Calories: 330 kcal
- Fat: 3.41 g
- Carbohydrates: 0.2 g
- Proteins: 20.9 g

Ingredients:

- 16 veal scallops
- Salt
- Ground pepper
- Garlic powder
- 2 eggs
- Breadcrumbs
- Extra virgin olive oil

Directions:

1. Put the beef scallops well spread, salt, and pepper. Add some garlic powder.
2. In a bowl, beat the eggs.
3. In another bowl, put the breadcrumbs.
4. Pass the Beef scallops for the beaten egg and then for the breadcrumbs.
5. Spray with extra virgin olive oil on both sides.
6. Put a batch in the basket of the air fryer. Do not pile the scallops too much.
7. Select 180°C and 15 minutes. From time to time, shake the basket so that the scallops move.
8. When finishing that batch, put the next one and so on until you finish with everyone, usually 4 or 5 scallops enter per batch.

CHEESY BEEF PASEÍLLO

Preparation Time: 9 minutes

Cooking Time: 23 minutes

Servings: 15

Nutritional values:

- Calories: 225 kcal
- Fat: 3.41 g
- Carbohydrates: 0 g
- Proteins: 20.9 g

Ingredients:

- 1-2 tbsp. olive oil
- 2 pounds lean ground beef
- ½ chopped onion
- 2 cloves garlic, minced
- ½ tbsp. Adobo seasoning
- 2 tsp. dried oregano
- 1 packet optional seasoning
- 2 tbsp. chopped cilantro

- ¼ cup grated cheese
- 15 dough disks
- 15 slices yellow cheese

Directions:

1. In a large skillet over medium-high heat, heat the oil. Once the oil has warmed, add the meat, onions, and Adobo seasoning.

2. Brown veal, about 6–7 minutes. Drain the ground beef. Add the remaining seasonings and cilantro. Cook an additional minute. Add grated cheese, if desired. Melt the cheese.

3. On each dough disk, add a slice of cheese to the center and add 3-4 tbsp. of the meat mixture over the slice of cheese. Fold over the dough disk and with a fork, fold the edges and set it aside.

4. Preheat the air fryer to 370°F for 3 minutes.

5. Once three minutes have passed, spray the air fryer pan with cooking spray and add 3–4 cupcakes to the basket. Close the basket, set it to 370°F, and cook for 7 minutes. After 7 minutes, verify it. Cook up to 3 additional minutes, or the desired level of sharpness, if desired.

6. Repeat until finished.

PORK HEAD CHOPS WITH VEGETABLES

Preparation Time: 9 minutes

Cooking Time: 24 minutes

Servings: 4

Nutritional values:

- Calories: 106 kcal
- Fat: 3.41 g
- Carbohydrates: 0 g
- Proteins: 20.9 g

Ingredients:

- 4 pork head chops
- 2 red tomatoes
- 1 large green pepper
- 4 mushrooms
- 1 onion
- 4 slices of cheese

- Salt
- Ground pepper
- Extra virgin olive oil

Directions:

1. Put the four chops on a plate and salt and pepper.
2. Put two of the chops in the air fryer basket.
3. Place tomato slices, cheese slices, pepper slices, onion slices and mushroom slices. Add some threads of oil.
4. Take the air fryer and select 180°C, 20 minutes.
5. Check that the meat is well made and take out.
6. Repeat the same operation with the other two pork chops.

AIR-FRIED FISH NUGGETS

Preparation Time: 15 minutes

Cooking Time: 15 minutes

Servings: 4

Nutritional values:

- Calories: 184 kcal
- Fat: 3 g
- Carbohydrates: 10 g
- Proteins: 19 g

Ingredients:

- 2 cups (skinless) fish fillets in cubes:
- 1 egg, beaten
- 5 tbsp. flour
- 5 tbsp. water
- Kosher salt and pepper to taste
- Breadcrumbs mix

- 1 tbsp. smoked paprika
- ¼ cup whole wheat breadcrumbs
- 1 tbsp. garlic powder

Directions:

1. Season the fish cubes with kosher salt and pepper.
2. In a bowl, add flour and gradually add water, mixing as you add.
3. Then mix in the egg. And keep mixing but do not over mix.
4. Coat the cubes in batter, then in the breadcrumb mix. Coat well
5. Place the cubes in a baking tray and spray with oil.
6. Let the air fryer preheat to 200°C.
7. Place cubes in the air fryer and cook for 12 minutes or until well cooked and golden brown.
8. Serve with salad greens.

GARLIC ROSEMARY GRILLED PRAWNS

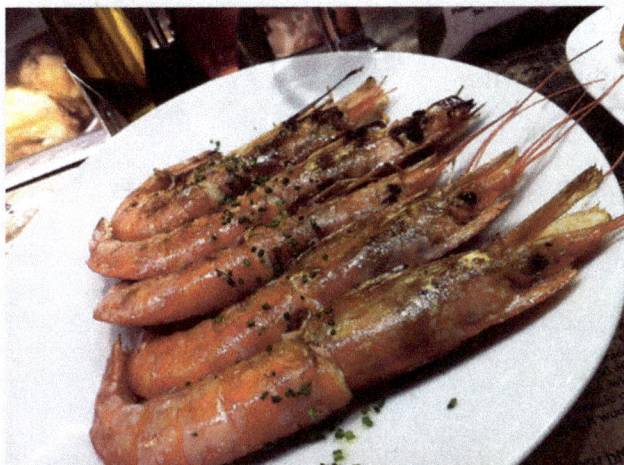

Preparation Time: 5 minutes

Cooking Time: 11 minutes

Servings: 2

Nutritional values:

- Calories: 194 kcal
- Fat: 10 g
- Carbohydrates: 12 g
- Proteins: 26 g

Ingredients:

- Melted butter: ½ tbsp.
- Green capsicum: slices
- Eight prawns
- Rosemary leaves
- Kosher salt& freshly ground black pepper
- 3-4 cloves of minced garlic

Directions:

1. In a bowl, mix all the ingredients and marinate the prawns in it for at least 60 minutes or more
2. Add two prawns and two slices of capsicum on each skewer.
3. Let the air fryer preheat to 180 C.
4. Cook for 5-6 minutes. Then change the temperature to 200 C and cook for another minute.
5. Serve with lemon wedges.

AIR-FRIED CRUMBED FISH

Preparation Time: 10 minutes

Cooking Time: 12 minutes

Servings: 2

Nutritional values:

- Calories: 254 kcal
- Fat: 12.7 g
- Carbohydrates: 10.2 g
- Proteins: 15.5 g

Ingredients:

- Four fish fillets
- 4 tbsp. olive oil
- 1 egg beaten
- ¼ cup whole wheat breadcrumbs

Directions:

1. Let the air fryer preheat to 180 C.

2. In a bowl, mix breadcrumbs with oil. Mix well

3. First, coat the fish in the egg mix (egg mix with water), then in the breadcrumb mix. Coat well

4. Place in the air fryer, let it cook for 10-12 minutes.

5. Serve hot with salad green and lemon.

CRISPY CHICKEN FILLETS

Preparation Time: 12 minutes

Cooking Time: 18 minutes

Servings: 3

Nutritional values:

- Calories: 142 kcal
- Fat: 5 g
- Carbohydrates: 3 g
- Proteins: 23 g

Ingredients:

- 2 tbsp. vegetable oil
- 2 large eggs (whisked)
- 13 ounces chicken fillets
- 9 tbsp. breadcrumbs
- 1 tsp. freshly ground black pepper

- 3 and ½ ounces all-purpose flour
- ½ a tsp. kitchen salt

Directions:

1. Turn on your Air Fryer and preheat to 340°F.
2. Then add the kitchen salt, ground black pepper, and vegetable oil to the breadcrumbs and combine by mixing totally.
3. Get two shallow bowls and transfer the whisked eggs into one and the all-purpose flour in the other. Dip the chicken into the flour bowl, dust the chicken to get rid of surplus flour, and then dip the flour-coated chicken into the whisked eggs. Coat each fillet completely with breadcrumbs subsequently.
4. Take out the fry basket and lay the chicken fillets inside.
5. Cook fillets for 12 minutes and then step-up heat to 400°F, and continue cooking for an additional 5 minutes till fillets turn golden.

JERK STYLE CHICKEN WINGS

Preparation Time: 10 minutes

Cooking Time: 30 minutes

Servings: 3

Nutritional values:

- Calories: 240 kcal
- Fat: 15 g
- Carbohydrates: 5 g
- Proteins: 19 g

Ingredients:

- 1 g ground thyme
- 1 g dried rosemary
- 2 g allspice
- 4 g ground ginger
- 3 g garlic powder
- 2 g onion powder

- 1 g cinnamon
- 2 g paprika
- 2 g chili powder
- 1 g nutmeg
- Salt to taste
- 30 ml vegetable oil
- 0.5 - 1 kg (2 lb.) chicken wings
- 1 lime, juice

Directions:

1. Select Preheat, set the temperature to 200°C, and press Start/Pause.
2. Combine all spices and oil in a bowl to create a marinade.
3. Mix the chicken wings in the marinade until they are well covered.
4. Place the chicken wings in the preheated air fryer.
5. Select Chicken and press Start/Pause. Be sure to shake the baskets in the middle of cooking.
6. Remove the wings and place them on a serving plate.
7. Squeeze fresh lemon juice over the wings and serve.

ITALIAN CHICKEN

Preparation Time: 10 minutes

Cooking Time: 30 minutes

Servings: 4

Nutritional values:

- Calories: 272 kcal
- Fat: 9 g
- Carbohydrates: 37 g
- Proteins: 23 g

Ingredients:

- 5 chicken thighs
- 1 tbsp. olive oil
- ¼ cup parmesan; grated
- ½ cup sun-dried tomatoes
- 2 garlic cloves; minced
- 1 tbsp. thyme; chopped.
- ½ cup heavy cream
- 3/4 cup chicken stock

- 1 tsp. red pepper flakes; crushed
- 2 tbsp. basil; chopped
- Salt and black pepper to the taste

Directions:

1. Season chicken with salt and pepper, rub with half of the oil, place in your preheated air fryer at 350°F and cook for 4 minutes.

2. Meanwhile, preheat the pan with the rest of the oil over medium-high heat, add thyme, garlic, pepper flakes, sun-dried tomatoes, heavy cream, stock, parmesan, salt, and pepper; stir, then simmer, take off heat and transfer the dish that fits your air fryer.

3. Add chicken thighs on top, introduce in your air fryer and cook at 320°F for 12 minutes. Divide among plates and serve with basil sprinkled on top.

CHICKEN WINGS

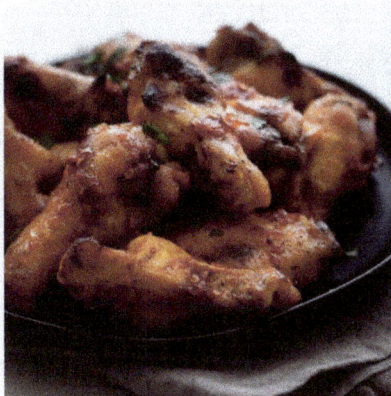

Preparation Time: 10 minutes

Cooking Time: 1 hour and 30 minutes

Servings: 4

Nutritional values:

- Calories: 240 kcal
- Fat: 16 g
- Carbohydrates: 4 g
- Proteins: 20 g

Ingredients:

- 3 pounds chicken wing parts, pastured

- 1 tbsp. old bay seasoning
- 1 tsp. lemon zest
- 3/4 cup potato starch
- ½ cup butter, unsalted, melted

Directions:

1. Switch on the air fryer, insert fryer basket, grease it with olive oil, then shut with its lid, set the fryer at 360°F and preheat for 5 minutes.

2. Meanwhile, pat dry chicken wings and then place them in a bowl.

3. Stir together seasoning and starch, add to chicken wings, and stir well until evenly coated.

4. Open the fryer, add the chicken wings in a single layer, close with its lid and cook for 35 minutes, shaking every 10 minutes.

5. Then switch the temperature of air fryer to 400°F and continue air frying the chicken wings for 10 minutes or until nicely golden brown and cooked, shaking every 3 minutes.

6. When the air fryer beeps, open its lid, transfer chicken wings onto a serving plate, and cook the remaining wings in the same manner.

7. Whisk together melted butter and lemon zest until blended and serve it with the chicken wings.

CHICKEN TENDERS

Preparation Time: 5 minutes

Cooking Time: 10 minutes

Servings: 2

Nutritional values:

- Calories: 112 kcal
- Fat: 6.2 g
- Carbohydrates: 7.1 g
- Proteins: 7 g

Ingredients:

- 1/8 cup almond flour
- 12 ounces chicken breasts, pastured
- ½ tsp. ground black pepper
- ¾ tsp. salt
- 1.2 ounces panko bread crumbs
- 1 egg white, pastured

Directions:

1. Switch on the air fryer, insert fryer basket, grease it with olive oil, then shut with its lid, set the fryer at 350°F and preheat for 5 minutes.

2. Meanwhile, season the chicken with salt and black pepper on both sides and then evenly coat it with flour.

3. Crack the egg, whisk until blended, dip the coated chicken in it and then coat with bread crumbs.

4. Open the fryer, add chicken in it, close with its lid and cook for 10 minutes until nicely golden and cooked, turning the chicken halfway through the frying.

5. When the air fryer beeps, open its lid, transfer chicken onto a serving plate and serve.

CHICKEN NUGGETS

Preparation Time: 10 minutes

Cooking Time: 24 minutes

Servings: 4

Nutritional values:

- Calories: 312 kcal
- Fat: 15 g
- Carbohydrates: 9 g
- Proteins: 33.6 g

Ingredients:

- 1-pound chicken breast, pastured
- ¼ cup coconut flour
- 6 tbsp. toasted sesame seeds
- ½ tsp. ginger powder
- 1/8 tsp. sea salt
- 1 tsp. sesame oil
- 4 egg whites, pastured

Directions:

1. Switch on the air fryer, insert fryer basket, grease it with olive oil, then shut with its lid, set the fryer at 400°F and preheat for 10 minutes.

2. Meanwhile, cut the chicken breast into 1-inch pieces, pat them dry, place the chicken pieces in a bowl, sprinkle with salt, oil and toss until well coated.

3. Place flour in a large plastic bag, add ginger and chicken, seal the bag, and turn it upside down to coat the chicken with flour evenly.

4. Place egg whites in a bowl, whisk well, then add coated chicken and toss until well coated.

5. Place sesame seeds in a large plastic bag, add chicken pieces in it, seal it, and turn it upside down to coat the chicken with sesame seeds evenly.

6. Open the fryer, add chicken nuggets in it in a single layer, spray with oil, close with its lid and cook for 12 minutes until nicely golden and cooked, turning the chicken nuggets and spraying with oil halfway through.

7. When the air fryer beeps, open its lid, transfer chicken nuggets onto a serving plate and fry the remaining chicken nuggets in the same manner.

8. Serve straight away.

CHICKEN MEATBALLS

Preparation Time: 5 minutes

Cooking Time: 26 minutes

Servings: 4

- **Nutritional values:**
- Calories: 223 kcal
- Carbohydrates: 3 g
- Proteins: 20 g
- Fat: 14 g

Ingredients:

- 1-pound ground chicken
- 2 green onions, chopped
- ¾ tsp. ground black pepper
- ¼ cup shredded coconut, unsweetened
- 1 tsp. salt
- 1 tbsp. hoisin sauce
- 1 tbsp. soy sauce
- ½ cup cilantro, chopped

- 1 tsp. Sriracha sauce
- 1 tsp. sesame oil

Directions:

1. Switch on the air fryer, insert fryer basket, grease it with olive oil, then shut with its lid, set the fryer at 350°F and preheat for 5 minutes.
2. Meanwhile, place all the ingredients in a bowl, stir until well mixed and then shape the mixture into meatballs, 1 tsp. of chicken mixture per meatball.
3. Open the fryer, add chicken meatballs in a single layer, close with its lid and then spray with oil.
4. Cook the chicken meatballs for 10 minutes, flipping the meatballs halfway through, and then continue cooking for 3 minutes until golden.
5. When the air fryer beeps, open its lid, transfer chicken meatballs onto a serving plate and then cook the remaining meatballs in the same manner.
6. Serve straight away.

AIR-FRIED AVOCADO WEDGES

Preparation Time: 3 minutes

Cooking Time: 10 minutes

Servings: 2

Nutritional values:

- Calories: 302 kcal
- Fat: 17.3 g
- Carbohydrates: 37.2 g
- Proteins: 8.3 g

Ingredients:

- ¼ cup flour
- ½ tsp. black pepper (ground)
- ¼ tsp. salt
- 1 tsp. water
- 1 ripe avocado (cut in eight slices)

- ½ cup bread crumbs
- 1 serving cooking spray

Directions:

1. Heat your air fryer at 200°C.
2. Combine pepper, salt, and flour in a bowl. Place water in another bowl.
3. Take a shallow dish and spread the bread crumbs.
4. Coat the avocado slices in a flour mixture and dip them in water.
5. Coat the slices in bread crumbs. Make sure both sides are evenly coated.
6. Use a cooking spray for misting the slices of avocado.
7. Cook the coated slices of avocado for four minutes. Flip the slices and cook again for three minutes.
8. Serve hot.

CRUNCHY GRAINS

Preparation Time: 9 minutes

Cooking Time: 16 minutes

Servings: 4

Nutritional values:

- Calories: 71 kcal
- Fat: 3.2 g
- Carbohydrates: 34.4 g
- Proteins: 5.8 g

Ingredients:

- 3 cups whole grains (cooked)
- ½ cup peanut oil

Directions:

1. Use a paper towel for removing excess moisture from the grains.

2.	Toss the grains in oil.

3.	Add the coated grains in the basket of the air fryer. Cook for ten minutes. Toss the grains and cook again for five minutes.

BUFFALO CHICKPEAS

Preparation Time: 14 minutes

Cooking Time: 15 minutes

Servings: 2

Nutritional values:

- Calories: 172 kcal
- Fat: 1.4 g
- Carbohydrates: 31.6 g
- Proteins: 7.2 g

Ingredients:

- 1 can chickpeas (rinsed)
- 2 tbsp. buffalo wing sauce
- 1 tbsp. ranch dressing mix (dry)

Directions:

1. Heat your air fryer at 175°C.

2. Use paper towels for removing excess moisture from the chickpeas.

3. Transfer the chickpeas to a bowl and add the wing sauce. Add the dressing mix and combine well.

4. Cook the chickpeas in the air fryer for eight minutes. Shake the basket and cook for five minutes.

5. Let the chickpeas sit for two minutes.

6. Serve warm.

EASY FALAFEL

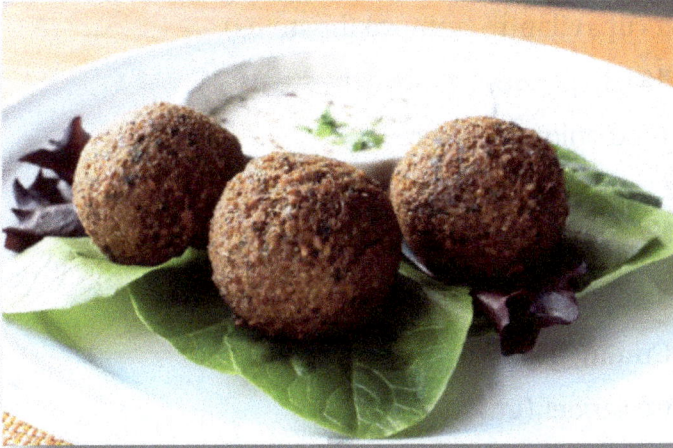

Preparation Time: 6 minutes

Cooking Time: 34 minutes

Servings: 15

Nutritional values:

- Calories: 57.9 kcal
- Fat: 1.4 g
- Carbohydrates: 8.9 g
- Proteins: 3.2 g

Ingredients:

- 1 cup garbanzo beans
- 2 cups cilantro (remove the stems)
- ¾ cup parsley (remove the stems)
- 1 red onion (quartered)
- One garlic clove
- 2 tbsp. chickpea flour
- 1 tbsp. each
- Cumin (ground)
- Coriander (ground)
- Sriracha sauce
- 1 tsp. black pepper and salt (for seasoning)
- ½ tsp. each
- Baking soda
- Baking powder
- 1 serving cooking spray

Directions:

1. Soak the beans in cool water for one day. Rub the beans and remove the skin. Rinse in cold water and use paper towels to remove excess moisture.

2. Add cilantro, beans, onion, parsley, and garlic in a blender. Blend the ingredients until paste forms.

3. Transfer the blended paste to a bowl and add coriander, flour, sriracha, cumin, pepper, and salt. Mix well. Let the mixture sit for twenty minutes.

4. Add baking soda and baking powder to the mixture. Mix well.

5. Make fifteen balls from the mixture and flatten them using your hands for making patties.

6. Use a cooking spray for greasing the falafel patties.

7. Cook them for ten minutes.

8. Serve warm.

MINI CHEESE AND BEAN TACOS

Preparation Time: 9 minutes

Cooking Time: 10 minutes

Servings: 12

Nutritional values:

- Calories: 229 kcal
- Fat: 10.4 g
- Carbohydrates: 20.2 g
- Proteins: 11.3 g

Ingredients:

- 1 can refried beans
- 1 ounce taco seasoning mix
- 12 slices American cheese (halved)
- 12 tortillas
- 1 serving cooking spray

Directions:

1. Place the beans in a medium-sized bowl. Add the seasoning mix. Combine well.

2. Place one cheese piece in the center of each tortilla. Take one tbsp. of the bean mix and add it over the cheese. Add another cheese piece over the beans. Fold the tortillas in half. Gently press with your hands for sealing the ends.

3. Use a cooking spray for spraying the tacos.

4. Cook the tacos for three minutes. Turn the tacos and cook again for three minutes

5. Serve hot.

GREEN BEANS AND SPICY SAUCE

Preparation Time: 7 minutes

Cooking Time: 29 minutes

Servings: 4

Nutritional values:

- Calories: 460.2 kcal
- Fat: 30.6 g
- Carbohydrates: 34.4 g
- Proteins: 5.7 g

Ingredients:

- 1 cup beer
- 1 and a half cup flour
- 2 tsps. salt
- ½ tsp. black pepper (ground)
- 12 ounces green beans (trimmed)

For the sauce:

- 1 cup ranch dressing
- 2 tsps. sriracha sauce
- 1 tsp. horseradish

Directions:

- Mix flour, beer, pepper, and salt in a mixing bowl. Add the beans in the batter and coat well. Shake off extra batter.
- Line the air fryer basket with parchment paper. Add the beans and cook for 20 minutes. Shake in between.
- Combine sriracha sauce, ranch dressing, and horseradish together in a bowl.
- Serve the beans with sauce by the side.

CHEESY SUGAR SNAP PEAS

Preparation Time: 5 minutes

Cooking Time: 13 minutes

Servings: 4

Nutritional values:

- Calories: 72 kcal
- Fat: 3.3 g
- Carbohydrates: 8.9 g
- Proteins: 5.7 g

Ingredients:

- ½ pound sugar snap peas
- 1 tsp. olive oil
- ¼ cup bread crumbs
- ½ cup parmesan cheese
- Pepper and salt (for seasoning)
- 2 tbsp. garlic (minced)

Directions:

1. Remove the stem from each pea pod. Rinse the peas and drain the water.

2. Toss the peas with bread crumbs, olive oil, pepper, salt, and half of the cheese.

3. Cook the peas in the air fryer for four minutes at 175°C.

4. Add minced garlic and cook again for five minutes.

5. Serve the peas with the remaining cheese from the top.

KIWI CHIPS

Preparation Time: 5 minutes

Cooking Time: 45 minutes

Servings: 6

Nutritional values:

- Calories: 110 kcal
- Fat: 1.1 g
- Carbohydrates: 26.3 g
- Proteins: 2.1 g

Ingredients:

- 1 kg kiwi
- ½ tsp. cinnamon (ground)
- ¼ tsp. nutmeg (ground)

Directions:

1. Slice the kiwi thinly. Keep them in a bowl.

2.   Sprinkle nutmeg and cinnamon from the top. Toss for mixing.

3.   Preheat the air fryer at 165°C.

4.   Cook the kiwi in the air fryer for half an hour. Make sure you shake the basket halfway.

5.   Let the chips cool down in the basket for fifteen minutes.

6.   Cool before serving.

APPLE CRISP

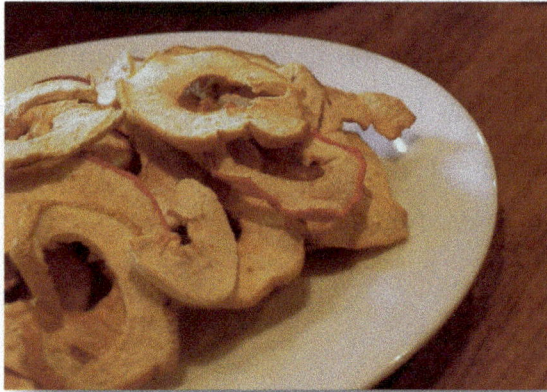

Preparation Time: 9 minutes

Cooking Time: 20-25 minutes

Servings: 2

Nutritional values:

- Calories: 341 kcal
- Proteins: 3.9 g
- Carbohydrates: 60.5 g
- Fat: 12.3 g

Ingredients:

- 2 apples (chopped)
- 1 tsp. each
- Lemon juice
- Cinnamon
- 2 tbsp. brown sugar

For the topping:

- 3 tbsp. flour
- 2 tbsp. brown sugar
- ½ tsp. salt
- 4 tbsp. rolled oats
- 1 and a half tbsp. butter

Directions:

1. Heat your air fryer at 170°C. Use butter for greasing the basket.
2. Combine lemon juice, apples, cinnamon, and sugar together in a bowl.
3. Cook the mixture for fifteen minutes. Shake the basket and cook again for five minutes.
4. For the topping, mix sugar, flour, salt, butter, and oats. Use an electric mixer for mixing.
5. Scatter the topping over the cooked apples. Return the basket to the air fryer. Cook again for five minutes.

TASTY ORANGE CAKE

Preparation Time: 42 minutes

Cooking Time: 20 minutes

Servings: 12

Nutritional values:

- Calories: 175 kcal
- Fat: 21 g
- Carbohydrates: 9 g
- Proteins: 4 g

Ingredients:

- 6 eggs
- 1 orange
- 1 tbsp. vanilla extract
- 1 tbsp. baking powder
- 9 oz. flour
- 2 oz. sugar + 2 tbsp.

- 2 tbsp. orange zest
- 4 oz. cream cheese
- 4 oz. yogurt

Directions:

1. Hump orange in a food processor properly.
2. Put 2 tbsp. sugar, flour, vanilla extract, baking powder and throb properly.
3. Move mix into 2 springform pans, put in the fryer and cook at 330°F for 16 minutes.
4. Mix in cream cheese with yogurt and orange zest and the rest of the sugar in a bowl and turn properly.
5. Put one cake layer on a plate, half of the cream cheese blend, then the other cake layer and the remaining cream cheese blend.
6. Properly rub, slice.
7. Serve.

MACAROONS

Preparation Time: 10 minutes

Cooking Time: 8 minutes

Servings: 20

Nutritional values:

- Calories: 172 kcal
- Fat: 11 g
- Carbohydrates: 7 g
- Proteins: 3 g

Ingredients:

- 2 tbsp. sugar
- 4 egg whites
- 2 cup coconut
- 1 tbsp. vanilla extract

Directions:

1. Mix in egg whites with stevia in a bowl and whisk using a mixer.

2. Put the coconut and vanilla extract, beat again, get small balls out of the mix, put in the air fryer, and cook at 340°F for 8 minutes.

3. Serve cold.

LIME CHEESECAKE

Preparation Time: 4 hours and 14 minutes

Cooking Time: 5 minutes

Servings: 10

Nutritional values:

- Calories: 199 kcal
- Fat: 11 g
- Carbohydrates: 8 g
- Proteins: 5 g

Ingredients:

- 2 tbsp. butter
- 2 tbsp. sugar
- 4 oz. flour
- ¼ cup coconut
- For the filling:
- 1 lb. cream cheese
- Zest from 1 lime
- Juice form 1 lime

- 2 cups hot water
- 2 sachets lime jelly

Directions:

1. Mix coconut with flour, sugar, and butter in a bowl, turn properly and compress mix to the bottom of the pan.
2. Get hot water in a bowl, put jelly sachets, and turn till it melts.
3. Get cream cheese in a bowl, put the lime juice, zest, and jelly and beat properly.
4. Get mix on the crust, rub, put in the air fryer and cook at 300°F for 4 minutes.
5. Cool in the fridge for 4 hours
6. Serve.

AIR FRIED SUGAR-FREE CHOCOLATE SOUFFLÉ

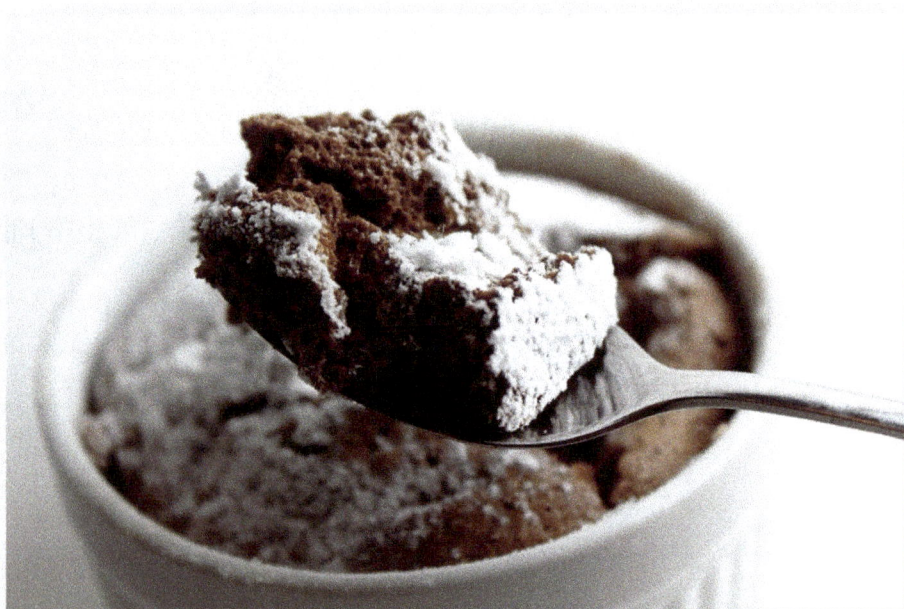

Preparation Time: 15 minutes

Cooking Time: 18 minutes

Servings: 2

Nutritional values:

- Calories: 288 kcal
- Fat: 24 g

- Carbohydrates: 5 g
- Proteins: 6 g

Ingredients:

- 1/3 cup milk
- 2 tbsp. butter soft to melt
- 1 tbsp. flour
- 2 tbsp. Splenda
- 1 egg yolk
- ¼ cup sugar-free chocolate chips
- 2 egg whites
- 1/2 tsp. cream of tartar
- 1/2 tsp. vanilla extract

Directions:

1. Grease the ramekins with spray oil or softened butter.
2. Sprinkle with any sugar alternative; make sure to cover them.
3. Let the air fryer preheat to 325–330°F
4. Melt the chocolate in a microwave-safe bowl. Mix every 30 seconds until fully melted.
5. Or use a double boiler method.

6. Melt the one and a half tbsp. of butter over low-medium heat. In a small-sized skillet.

7. Once the butter has melted, then whisk in the flour. Keep whisking until thickened. Then turn the heat off.

8. Add the egg whites with cream of tartar, with the whisk attachment, in a stand mixer, mix until peaks forms.

9. Meanwhile, combine the ingredients in a melted chocolate bowl, add the flour mixture and melted butter to chocolate, and blend. Add in the vanilla extract, egg yolks, and remaining sugar alternative.

10. Fold the egg white peaks gently with the ingredients into the bowl.

11. Add the mix into ramekins about 3/4 full of five-ounce ramekins

12. Let it bake for 12–14 minutes, or until done.

www.ingramcontent.com/pod-product-compliance
Lightning Source LLC
Chambersburg PA
CBHW050745030426
42336CB00012B/1660